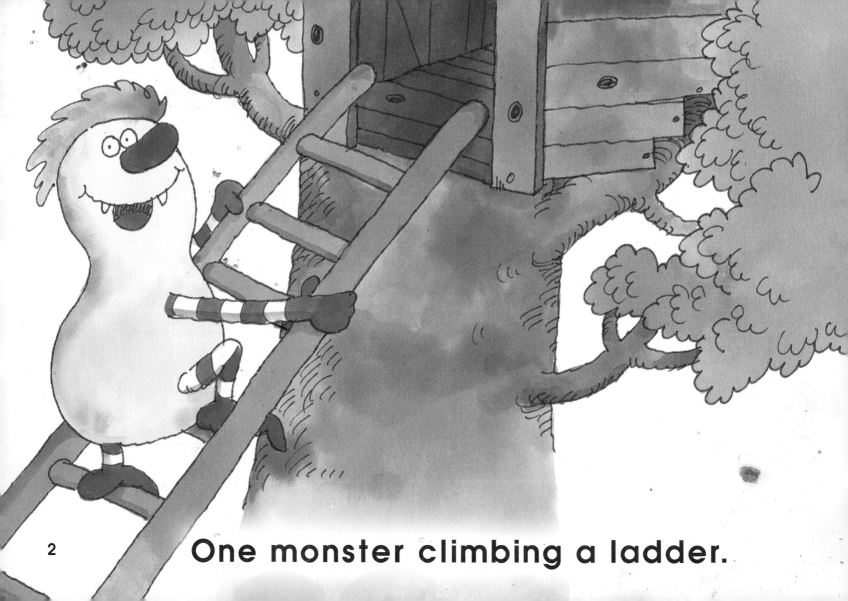

One monster climbing a ladder.

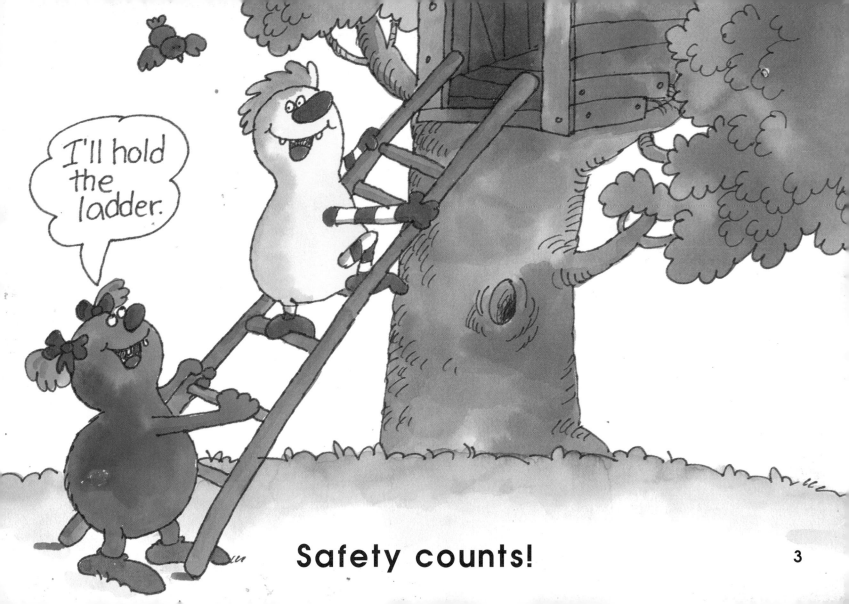

Safety counts!

**4** Two monsters cooking in the kitchen.

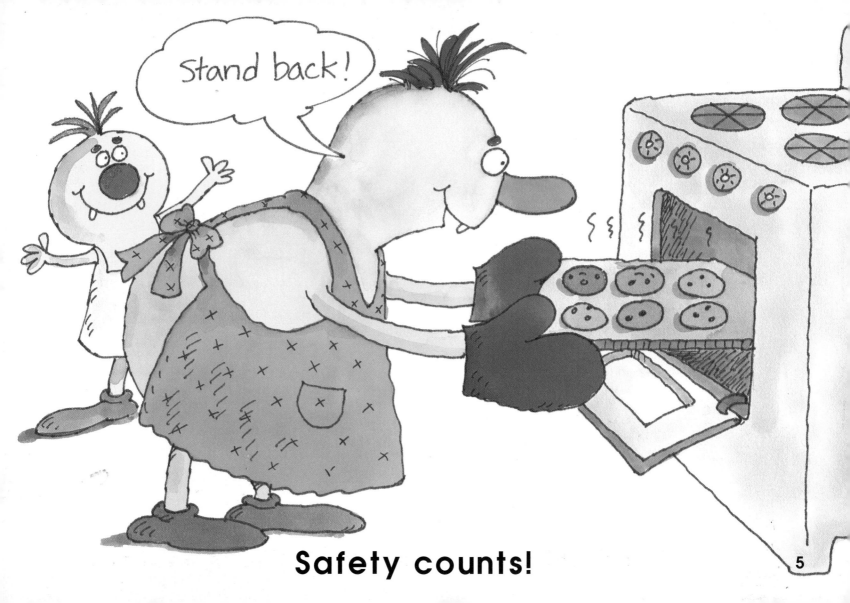

**Safety counts!**

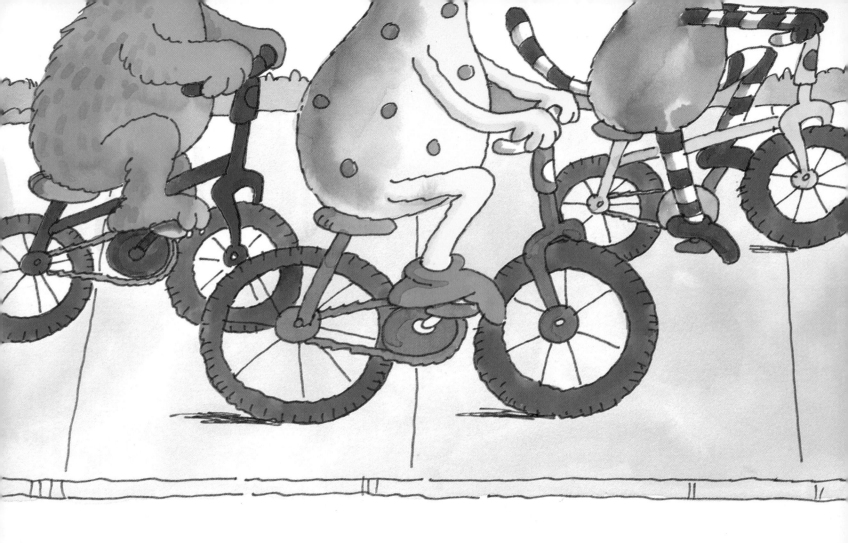

**Three monsters riding bicycles.**

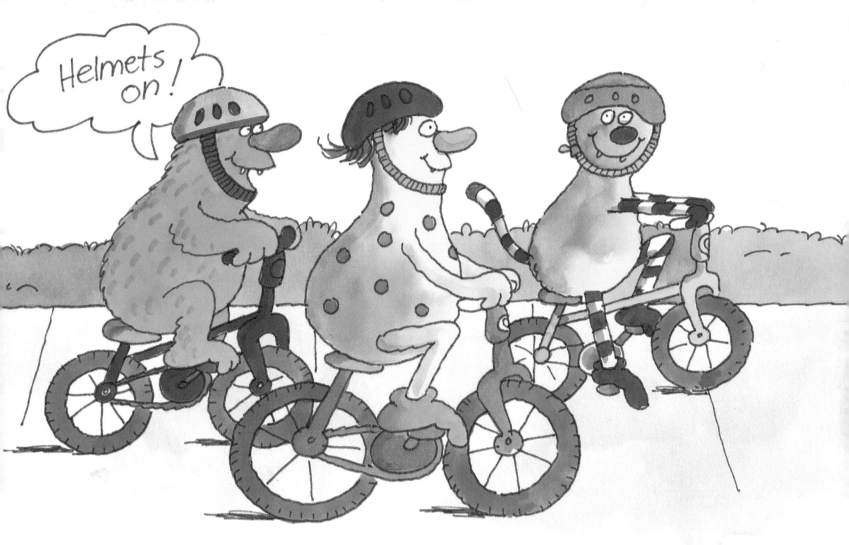

**Safety counts!**

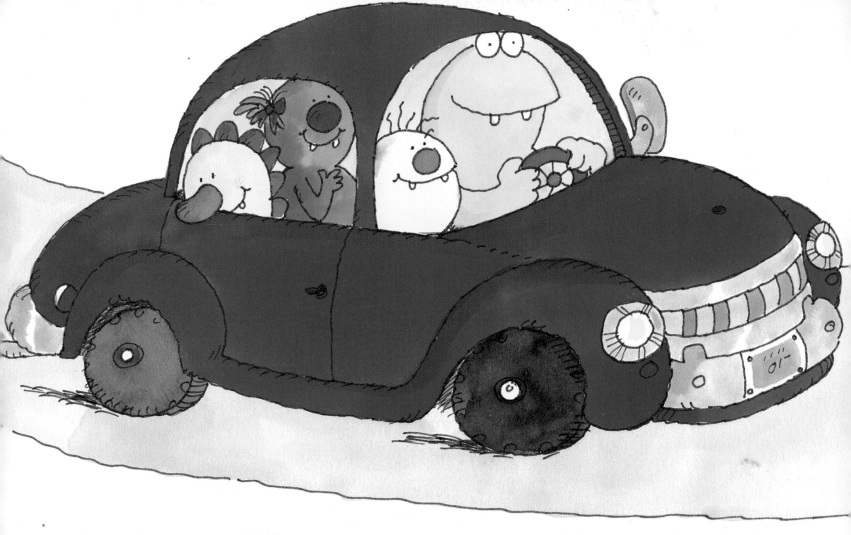

**Four monsters riding in a car.**

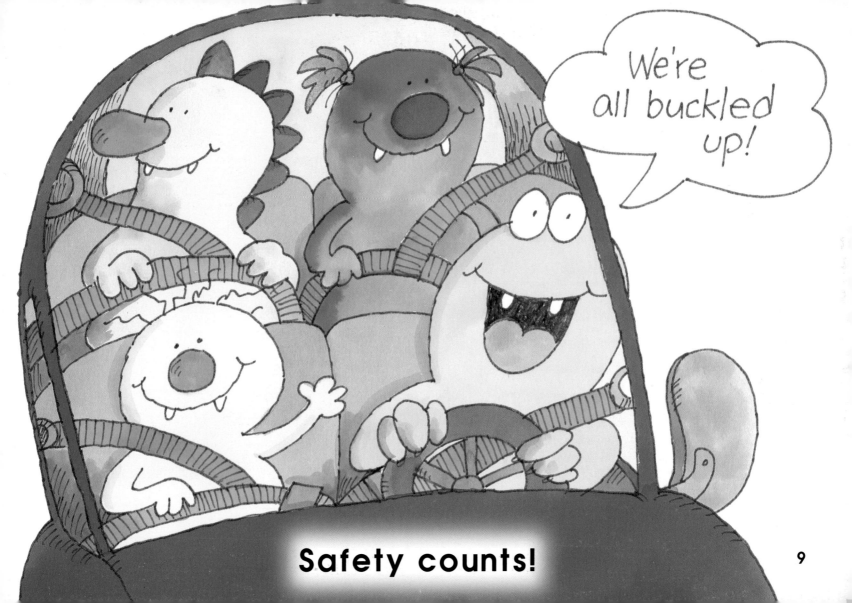

Safety counts!

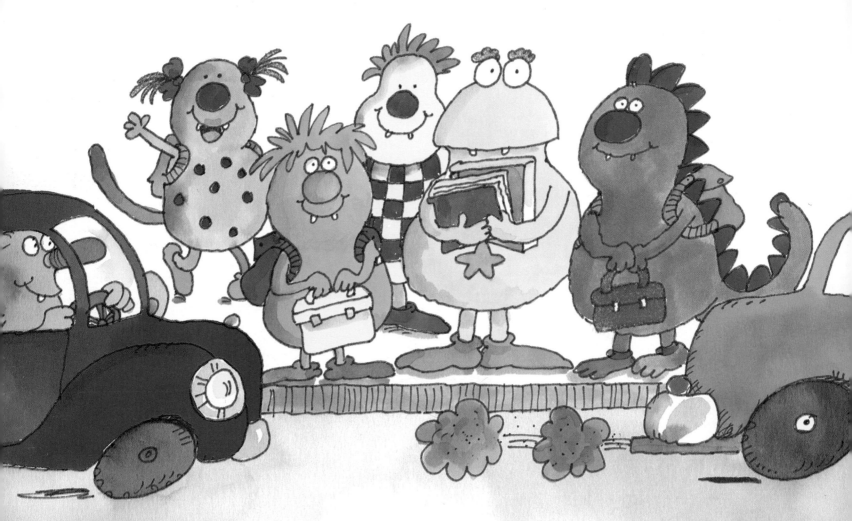

Five monsters crossing the street.

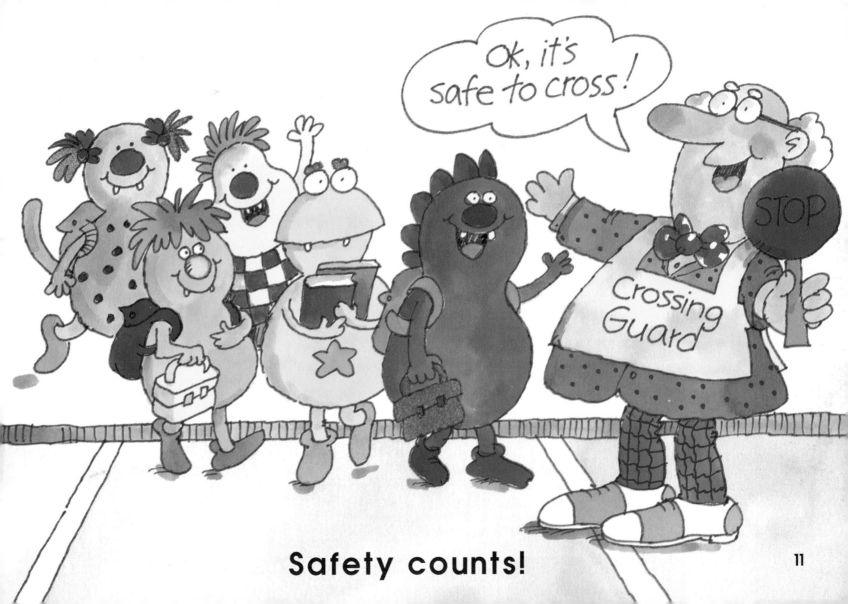

**Safety counts!**

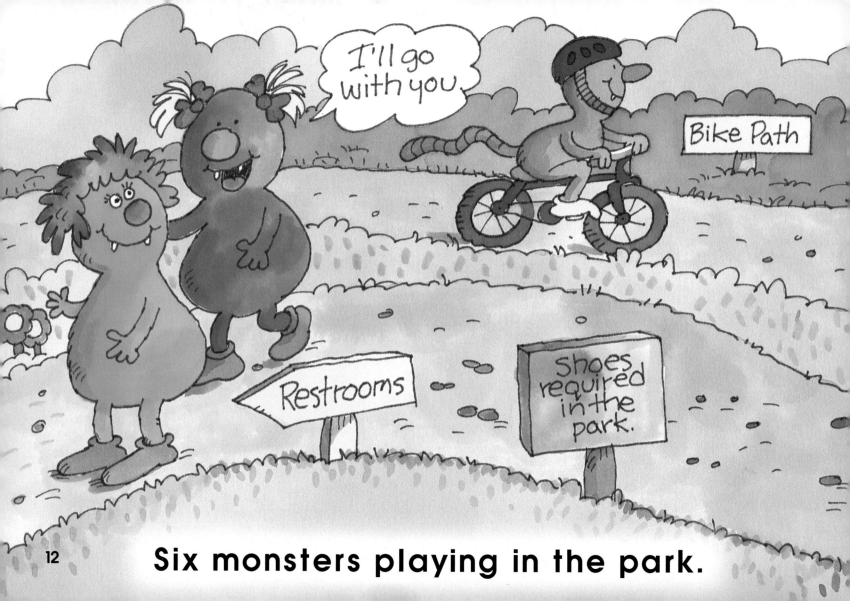

**Six monsters playing in the park.**

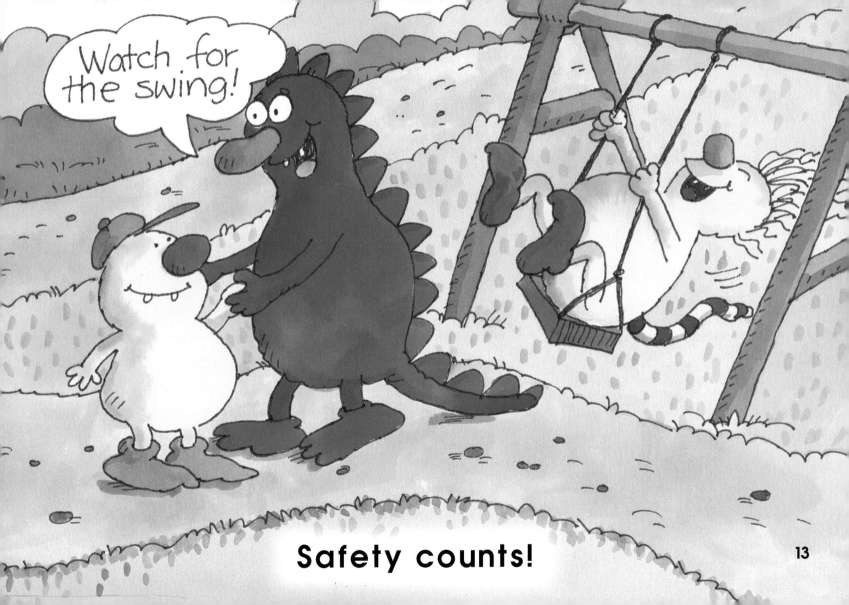

Safety counts!

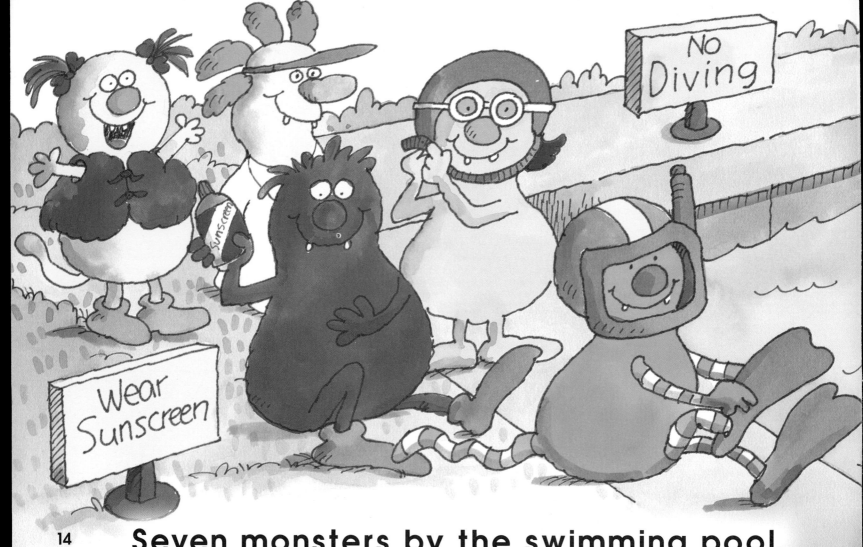

14 **Seven monsters by the swimming pool.**

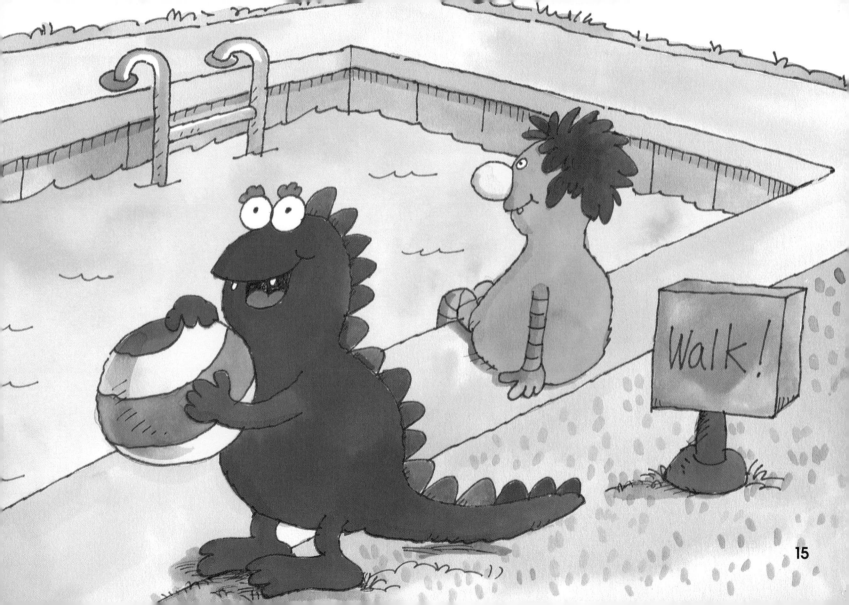

15

Safety counts!